RENAL DIET PLA

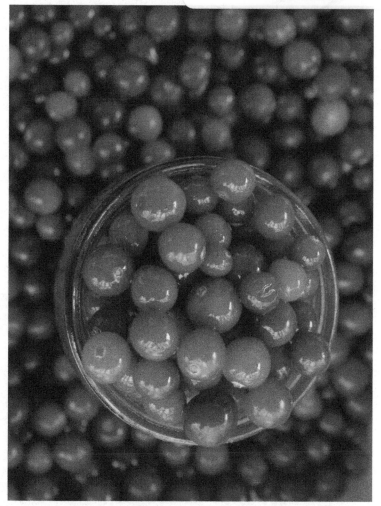

AVOID DIALYSIS AND MANAGE KIDNEY DISEASE WITH ONLY LOW SODIUM, LOW POTASSIUM, AND LOW PHOSPHORUS RECIPES!

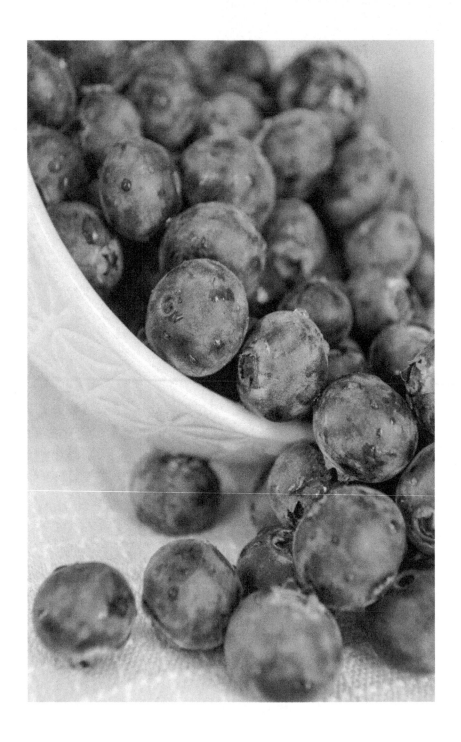

TABLE OF CONTENTS

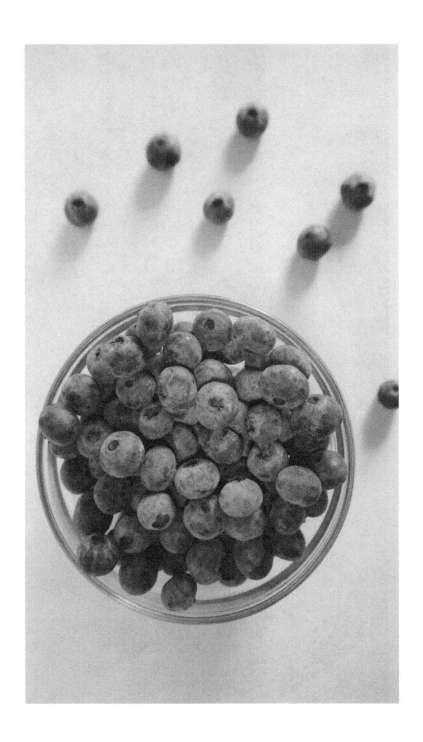

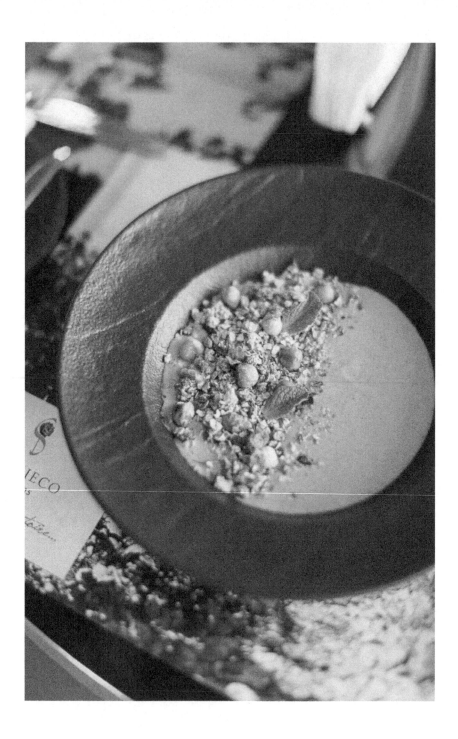

Introduction

At the very beginning, I would like to thank you for downloading this *"Renal Diet Plan and Cookbook! Avoid Dialysis and Manage Kidney Disease with Only Low Sodium, Low Potassium, and Low Phosphorus Recipes!"* This book is ideal for people with kidney disease and those who know someone (a friend, coworker, or a family member) with renal problems.

Kidney problems are complicated and require adequate management. Diet is an integral component of treatment for kidney disease and the best way to prevent potential complications such as dialysis or organ transplant.

A renal diet is easier to follow than most people think once you understand what to eat and avoid. The main purpose of this book is to introduce you to the world of renal diet and show some delicious yet healthy foods you can prepare easily in your kitchen.

Throughout the pages of this book, you'll learn more about kidney diseases and their causes, but also get valuable insight into renal diet, find out what you should eat and avoid, and so much more. Of course, the central component of the book is a cookbook with a 14-day renal diet plan, 60 recipes, and easy instructions.

The best thing about this cook is simplicity. All recipes are easy to make and feature accessible ingredients that won't be difficult to find, buy, and use. With our cookbook, you'll be able to improve the function of your kidneys and cut this risk of dialysis. This is also a great present for someone who has kidney disease and struggles to manage it. Sharing is caring!

Let's start our journey to healthier kidneys and happier life.

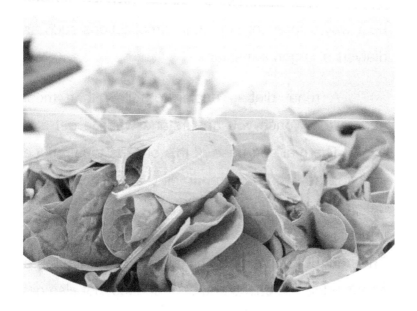

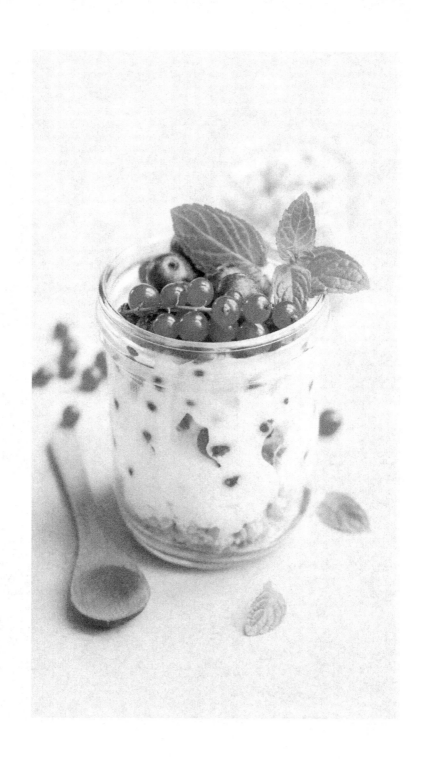

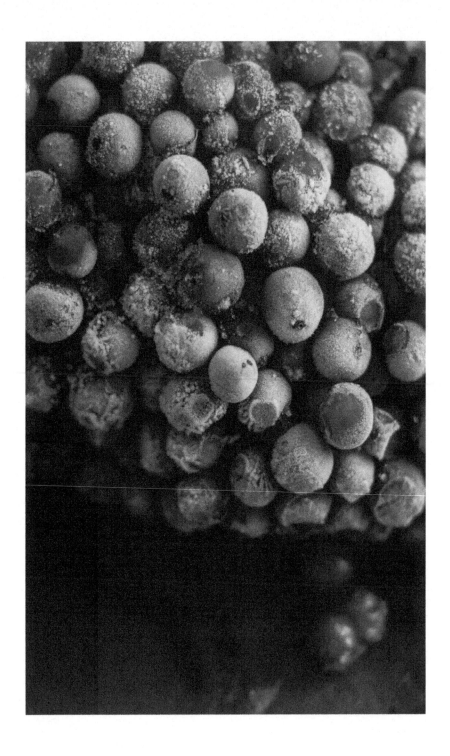

Chapter 1: What is Kidney Disease and How to Manage It?

The fact you are reading this book means that you are ready to make notable lifestyle adjustments for healthier kidneys and more effective disease management. Before we start cooking the amazing (and simple!) recipes from this book, it's important to learn a thing or two about kidneys and kidney disease.

Kidneys are two bean-shaped organs with important functions in the body. They maintain water balance and help expel waste. In humans, kidneys are about 10 cm (3.9 inches) long and are located underneath the diaphragm and right behind the peritoneum, large membrane in the abdominal cavity that supports and connects the internal organs. Each kidney in the body contains between 1,000,000 and 1,250,000 nephrons, functional units of the kidney. A nephron consists of tiny blood vessels, glomerulus, attached to a tubule. When blood enters the tiny blood vessels, it is filtered, and the remainder of fluid passes along the tubule where water and chemicals are either removed or added to the filtered fluid depending on the body's needs. The final product of this action is the urine.

Every 45 minutes, nephrons filter the whole five-quart water content of the blood or 160 quarts per day. Of this total amount, only one and a half quarts are excreted while the nephrons reabsorb the rest.

The most important functions of the kidneys are:

- Removal of waste products (toxins, excess salt, and urea) from the body

- Control of red blood cells production

- Removal of drugs from the body

- Production of an active form of vitamin D

- Balance of fluids in the body

- Release of hormones that regulate blood pressure

- Acid regulation

The proper function of the kidneys is vital for our health and wellbeing. These bean-shaped organs work a lot to keep us healthy, but they are prone to damage and disease, which can range in severity from one person to another.

What is Kidney Disease?

The term kidney disease refers to any damage to the kidneys and their inability to filter blood properly. Kidney disease is not a single condition, but an array of different problems that affect these organs. Unfortunately, kidney disease is largely underestimated on a global level. It is estimated that over 850 million people worldwide have some form of kidney disease, which is twice as much as diabetes and 20 times more than cancer prevalence.

The most common type of kidney disease in the world is chronic kidney disease (CKD), with an estimated prevalence of 11.8% in women and 10.4% in men. Figures also show that 5.3 to 10.5 million people worldwide require dialysis or kidney transplantation. About 13.3 million people experience acute kidney injury each year.

In the United States, approximately 15% of adults or 37 million people have chronic kidney disease. Unfortunately, nine out of 10 people with CKD don't even know they have it, while one in two people with low kidney function who are not on dialysis aren't aware they have CKD. Prevalence of CKD in the US women is 15% and 12% among men.

Types of Kidney Disease

As mentioned above, kidney disease is not a single condition but a term used to refer to a broad range of problems affecting the bean-shaped organs. Generally speaking, kidney diseases can be classified into:

- Acute kidney injury (AKI) – sudden damage to the kidneys that is usually short-term, but in some cases, it can progress to chronic kidney disease. Primary causes of AKI include obstruction to the urine leaving the kidney and damage to the kidney tissue caused by severe infection, medications, and radioactive dye

- Chronic kidney disease (CKD) – a long-term kidney problem that doesn't improve over time. A number of causes can contribute to CKD, including hypertension (high blood pressure), more about this in the next chapter. People of CKD are also at a higher risk of AKI and may also suffer from kidney failure, end-stage kidney disease, which requires dialysis or a kidney transplant

16

Now that you know categories to which kidney diseases are classified, here are some of the most common conditions that people may develop:

- Kidney stones – occur when minerals and other substances in the blood catalyze in the kidneys, thus forming a solid mass or stones. While they usually leave the body during urination passing a kidney stone can be quite painful

- Glomerulonephritis – inflammation of the glomeruli

- Polycystic kidney disease – a genetic disorder that induces the growth of multiple cysts on the kidneys. Cysts disrupt the function of these organs and may lead to kidney failure

- Urinary tract infections (UTIs) – bacterial infections are affecting any segment of the urinary system. The most common UTIs occur in urethra and bladder, but when not treated properly they may spread to the kidneys

- Lupus nephritis – kidney swelling and irritation caused by lupus, an autoimmune disease

- Kidney cancer – the most common type of kidney cancer is renal cell carcinoma and starts in the small filters in the kidneys

- Alport syndrome – a genetic condition indicated by kidney disease, hearing loss, and eye abnormalities

- Diabetic nephropathy – kidney damage that results from having diabetes

- Fabry disease – an inherited disorder resulting from the accumulation of globotriaosylceramide, a type of fat, in the cells. It can affect kidneys, skin, and heart

How to Manage Kidney Disease?

The actual treatment of kidney disease depends on multiple factors such as the underlying cause, type of the disease, severity of symptoms, and overall health of a patient. Some diseases can be treated successfully, but others do not have a cure. Before we go on, it's important to clarify this "have no cure" part. Just because there is no drug or other forms of treatment to eliminate the disease entirely, it doesn't mean there is nothing you can do about it. An adequate treatment approach can reduce the intensity of the symptoms, improve your quality of life, prevent the need for dialysis, and make you an overall healthier person.

Generally speaking, the treatment usually revolves around the measures to control symptoms, decrease the risk of complications, and slow down the progression of some specific kidney disease. Patients with kidney disease need to work closely with their doctor, who will recommend an adequate treatment approach for their condition and symptoms experienced.

Kidney disease oftentimes induces various complications that are treated with medications such as those for high blood pressure, anemia, high cholesterol levels, swelling, stronger bones. The most important thing to remember is that proper management of kidney disease also requires diet adjustment. In fact, your doctor will also recommend you should make some tweaks in your diet. That's the whole purpose of this book – to show you how easy it is to adopt a renal diet and make some super delicious foods along the way.

In cases when kidneys are unable to keep up with the clearance of waste and fluid on their own, and a patient develops near-complete kidney failure, end-stage kidney disease occurs. As mentioned above, at this point, it is necessary to undergo dialysis or organ transplant.

An important part of kidney disease treatment is lifestyle modification and the adoption of a kidney-friendly diet, which will be discussed further in this book.

Chapter 2: Causes and Symptoms of Kidney Disease

Kidneys may be small, but they do have important functions in the body. These bean-shaped organs work hard, but they may experience injuries and other problems that prevent them from functioning properly. But the question is what causes kidney disease and how to detect it? You'll get the answers in this chapter.

Causes and Risk Factors

What many of us are not aware of is that the cause of kidney disease doesn't necessarily have to occur in kidneys themselves. Problems affecting our overall health and wellbeing can also induce damage to the kidneys. In the same way, common health problems can also impair the function of these organs. The most frequent causes of kidney disease are hypertension and diabetes.

High blood pressure, which affects 75 million people in the US or one in three adults, can damage blood vessels in the kidney and thereby impair their function. In other words, damage to blood vessels in the kidneys due to hypertension doesn't allow them to remove wastes and extra fluid from your body. This leads to a vicious cycle as an accumulation of waste, and extra fluid increases blood pressure. Besides damaging filtering units in kidneys, high blood pressure can also reduce the flow of blood to these organs. As you're already aware, without a blood supply, organs cannot function properly.

About 30.3 million people or 9.4% of the population in the United States have diabetes which can cause a number of complications. Just like hypertension, diabetes also damages small blood vessels in the kidneys. As a result, the body retains more salt and water than it should. Moreover, diabetes also causes damage to the nerves in the body, which can make it difficult for you to empty the bladder. The pressure from a full bladder can back up and damage or injure kidneys. Let's also not forget the fact that if urine remains in the body for a long time, it can lead to an infection from the fast growth of bacteria and high blood sugar levels. Estimates show that 30% of patients with type 1 diabetes and 10% to 40% of people with type 2 diabetes will eventually experience kidney failure.

Besides diabetes and hypertension, other causes of kidney disease include:

- Infection

- Renal artery stenosis

- Heavy metal poisoning

- Lupus

- Some drugs

- Prolonged obstruction of the urinary tract from conditions such as kidney stones, enlarged prostate, some cancers

While everyone can develop kidney disease, some people are at a higher risk than others. Common risk factors for kidney disease include:

- Older age

- High blood pressure

- Diabetes

- Abnormal kidney structure

- Cardiovascular disease

- Family history of kidney disease

- Smoking

- Overweight and obesity

- Being of Native American, African American, and Asian American descent

Symptoms of Kidney Disease

Signs and symptoms of kidney disease don't appear suddenly, and they develop over time. Many people don't even know they have kidney disease until it reaches late stages because they are unable to identify some warning signs. Symptoms of kidney diseases may vary from one person to another as well as their severity. But generally speaking, the most common signs of kidney disease include:

- Nausea and vomiting

- Hypertension that is difficult to control

- Loss of appetite

- Shortness of breath

- Chest pain

- Weakness or fatigue

- Sleep disturbances

- Persistent itching

- Changes in how much a patient urinates

- Swollen feet and ankles

- Reduced mental sharpness

- Muscle cramps and twitching

- Blood in urine or foamy urine

It is worth mentioning that symptoms of kidney disease can be nonspecific as they are greatly influenced by causes of these conditions and underlying diseases.

Chapter 3: Renal Diet Overview

Kidney disease requires a proactive approach to reduce the intensity of symptoms and improve a patient's quality of life. Eating habits play a vital role in the management of kidney disease. Therefore, the most important thing you can do to manage your condition and prevent dialysis is to adopt a renal diet.

What is the Renal Diet?

A renal diet is defined as a diet that is low in protein, sodium, and phosphorus. This diet emphasizes the importance of limiting fluids and consuming high-quality proteins, but some patients may also need to decrease their intake of calcium and potassium. The main goal of the renal diet is to support kidney function and decrease the need for dialysis, but in order for it to work, one needs to adhere to it religiously. A renal diet is not a diet fad that comes and goes, and it's not a program one should follow for a few weeks. Instead, it's a way of life. Below you can see the breakdown of the most important components you need to monitor when on a renal diet.

Sodium

First, it's important to clarify that sodium is not a synonym for salt, as many people believe. Salt is just a compound of sodium and chloride. On the other hand, sodium is a mineral naturally present in many foods and important for body functions. In addition to potassium and chloride, sodium is an electrolyte meaning it helps control fluid levels in cells and tissues.

Sodium helps maintain blood pressure, regulates nerve function and muscle contraction, controls acid-base balance in the blood, among other things.

However, excessive levels of sodium are harmful to patients with kidney disease due to the fact these organs are unable to eliminate sodium and fluid from the body in an adequate manner.

As a result, fluid and sodium start accumulating and may cause a number of problems such as increased thirst, edema, hypertension, heart failure, and shortness of breath.

Phosphorus

27

Phosphorus is a mineral required for the maintenance and development of bones. This mineral also participates in the development of connective tissues, takes part in muscle movement, and so much more. Damaged kidneys don't remove excess phosphorus from the body. In turn, levels of this mineral accumulate and impair calcium balance, thus causing weak bones and calcium deposits in blood vessels.

Potassium

Potassium is an important mineral that participates in many functions, including muscle function, and it helps promote a healthy heartbeat. Like sodium, potassium is also necessary for fluid and electrolyte balance.

While potassium is needed for our health, patients with kidney disease do need to reduce the intake of this mineral. The reason is simple; when kidneys are damaged, they are not able to eliminate excess potassium out of the body. This causes a buildup of potassium and leads to other problems such as muscle weakness, heart attack, slow pulse, irregular heartbeat.

Through renal diet and recipes shown in this book, you will be able to reduce potassium intake and still improve your health and prevent potential complications that would arise with excess potassium levels.

Protein

Protein is one of the most important nutrients we need to consume on a daily basis. Generally speaking, protein is not a problem for people with healthy kidneys because it is eliminated out of the body with the help of renal proteins and filtering units. But people with kidney disease need to be cautious about how much protein they consume because their body doesn't remove this nutrient properly.

Fluid

People with kidney disease need to manage fluid intake, especially in later stages. The reason leads us back to the main function of the kidneys, which is to balance the fluid levels and help expel the waste. Impaired function of the bean-shaped organs causes fluid buildup as they are unable to remove it properly. For example, dialysis patients have reduced the output of urine, so a higher intake of

29

fluids can create unwanted and unnecessary pressure on the lungs and heart.

Why Do You Need a Renal Diet Plan?

It's not uncommon for people to wonder whether they really need a renal diet plan. But, if you have some kidney disease, you should definitely consider adopting this diet in order to improve your quality of life. The benefits of a renal diet plan are numerous and are scientifically confirmed. Studies show that diet plays a crucial role in patients with renal disease, and a slight increase in any component of diet can make a big difference in the pathogenesis of the disease. During the progression of CKD, the requirements and consumption of various nutrients change significantly. That's why it's important to see the doctor regularly and adhere to their instructions regarding diet and eating habits.

Here are some of many benefits and reasons to adopt a renal diet plan:

- Prevention of kidney stones

- Improved fluid balance

- Weight management

- Prevention of osteoporosis

- Healthier blood pressure

- Reduced risk of dialysis

- Slowed progression of kidney disease

- Improved function of kidneys e.g., to eliminate waste more effectively

- Protection of blood vessels

- Reduced buildup of fat

As you can see, the main advantage of the renal diet plan is that it works to enhance the function of the kidneys, but also to promote your overall health and wellbeing in order to prevent complications that would lead to dialysis and other problems. A diet specifically intended for people with kidney disease allows them to balance their fluid levels more effectively and allow filtering units in the kidneys to do their job.

Chapter 4: Foods to Eat and Avoid with Kidney Disease

In *Chapter 3*, we have established the importance of a renal diet and why you should include it in your lifestyle. Most people assume that it's difficult to follow the renal diet, but it's easier than you think. To get the best results (improved kidney function, reduced dialysis risk), it is important to learn more about diet in kidney disease. When you learn what to eat and avoid, it becomes a lot easier to adjust your eating habits. So, before we start cooking some delicious foods, we are going to go through the list of foods you should eat and definitely avoid when trying to manage kidney disease.

It's important to repeat that diet restrictions vary according to the stage of kidney disease. Renal diet usually involves limiting the consumption of potassium and sodium to 2000mg a day and lowering phosphorus intake to 1000mg per day.

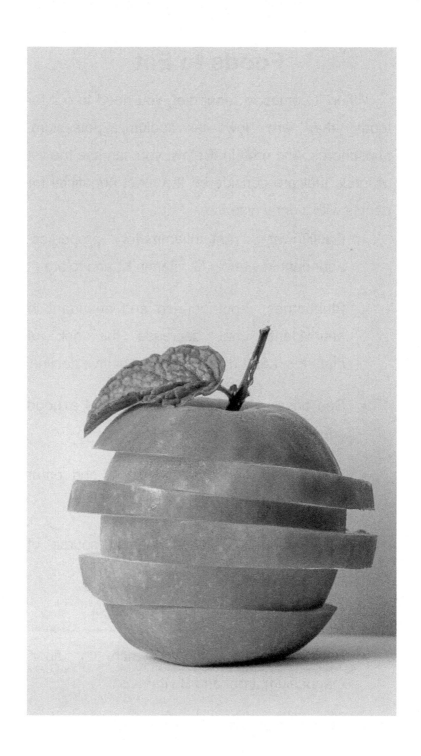

Foods to Eat

When it comes to renal diet, you need to opt for foods that are low in sodium, potassium, phosphorus, and protein. Below, you can see the list of foods that are considered the most beneficial for people with kidney disease:

- Cauliflower – anti-inflammatory properties, abundant in vitamin C, vitamin K, and folate

√ - Blueberries – nutrient-rich and abundant in antioxidants that decrease the risk of diabetes, heart disease, and cognitive decline

- Sea bass – high-quality protein and a good source of Omega-3 fatty acids

√ - Red grapes – rich in vitamin C and other valuable nutrients

√ - Egg whites – a kidney-friendly source of protein

√ - Garlic – a delicious alternative to salt

- Buckwheat – nutritious, rich in fiber, magnesium, iron, and B vitamins

√ - Olive oil – phosphorus-free

- Bulgur – kidney-friendly alternative to whole grains

- Cabbage – a great source of vitamin K, vitamin C, and B-complex vitamins

- Skinless chicken – contains less phosphorus, sodium, and potassium than chicken with skin on (remember, an adequate amount of protein is important for your health)

- Bell peppers – low in potassium

- Onions – sodium-free flavor for renal diet

- Arugula – nutrient-dense green vegetable low in potassium

- Macadamia nuts – low in phosphorus

- Radish – low in potassium and phosphorus

- Turnip – excellent replacement for high-potassium vegetables such as potatoes

- Pineapple – low potassium content

- Cranberries – contain nutrients that prevent bacteria from sticking to the lining of the bladder and urinary tract to cut the risk of infections

- Shiitake mushrooms – a plant-based meat substitute

√ • Apples – high in fiber and anti-inflammatory compounds

Foods to Avoid

In order to follow the renal diet that will support kidney function and not disrupt it, you may want to avoid consuming the following foods:

- Avocado – while they are healthy, avocadoes are abundant in potassium

✗ • Canned foods – contain high amounts of sodium

✗ • Whole-wheat bread – due to its phosphorus and potassium content

✗ • Brown rice – high in potassium and phosphorus

✗ • Bananas – abundant in potassium

✗ • Dairy – a natural source of phosphorus, potassium, protein

36

- X • Oranges (and OJ) – a rich source of potassium

- X • Processed meat – contain high amounts of salt

- X • Olives, pickles, and relish – too much salt

- X • Apricots – high in potassium

- X • Potatoes and sweet potatoes – contain high levels of potassium

- X • Tomatoes – high in potassium

- X • Instant, packaged, and premade meals – abundant in sodium

- • Spinach, beet greens, Swiss chard – contain high amounts of potassium

- X • Prunes, raisins, and dates – abundant in potassium

- X • Crackers, chips, pretzels, and other snacks – high in salt

NOTE: some foods such as potatoes and sweet potatoes can be leached or soaked to reduce potassium content.

Fluids and Juices for Healthy Kidneys

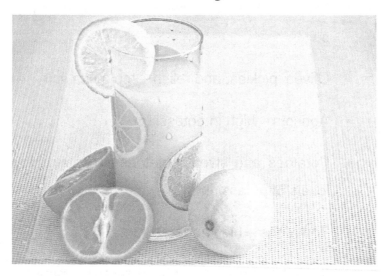

Management of kidney disease also requires paying attention to fluid intake and the things you drink. For example, you should definitely avoid soda, especially dark-colored cola. But, here are some drinks you should include in your lifestyle:

- Cranberry juice – beneficial for urinary and kidney health

- Lemon- and lime-based or other citrus juice – kidney stone prevention

- Water – allows kidneys to filter waste and toxins from the blood

- Stinging nettle tea – antioxidant-rich, reduces inflammation

Now that you know what to eat and avoid on the renal diet, it's time to start cooking. In the next chapters, you will see some of the best, easiest, and most delicious recipes that you can make.

Chapter 5: Breakfast

Breakfast is the most important meal of the day, and that doesn't change with kidney disease. People with kidney disease need to pay attention to the ingredients they use for their breakfasts. In this chapter, you're going to see how to have a super delicious breakfast with a renal diet.

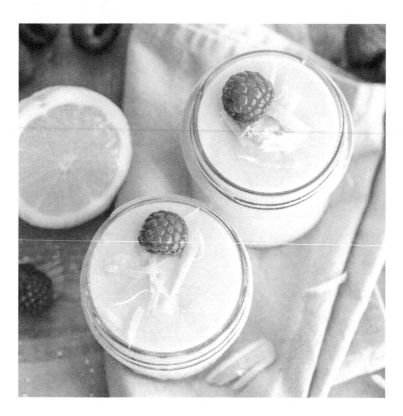

Day #1: Microwave Egg W
French Toast

This take on a French toast is simple, delicious, and hassle-free. It's a perfect breakfast option for busy mornings when you're in a hurry to get ready and go to work.

COOKING TIME: 5 MINUTES

INGREDIENTS FOR 1 SERVING

- Bread slice – 1

- Unsalted butter (softened) – 1tsp

- Egg white – ½ cup

- Sugar-free syrup – 2 tbsp

METHOD

- Spread butter over bread slice and cut it into cubes

- Place the cubes into a bowl and pour egg whites over bread

- Sprinkle a little bit of syrup on top

- Place the bowl into a microwave for 1 minute

- Use a fork or spoon to bring the uncooked egg to the surface

- Return to microwave for an additional minute

- Serve warm

NUTRITIONAL INFORMATION (per serving)

- Calories – 200

- Carbohydrate – 24g

- Protein – 15g

- Sodium – 415mg

- Potassium – 235mg

- Phosphorus – 54mg

- Dietary fiber – 0.7g

- Fat – 5g

Day #2: Blueberry Pancake

Everybody loves pancakes, and now you have the chance to make delicious yet kidney-friendly breakfast low in phosphorus.

COOKING TIME: 10 MINUTES

INGREDIENTS FOR 6 SERVINGS (12pancakes)

SERVING SIZE: 2 pancakes

- All-purpose flour (sifted) – 1 ½ cups

- Baking powder – 2tsp

- Sugar – 3tbsp

- Buttermilk – 1 cup

- No-salt margarine (melted) – 2tbsp

- Eggs (slightly beaten) – 2

- Blueberries – 1 cup

METHOD

- In a mixing bowl combine flour, baking powder, and sugar

43

- Make a little "hole" in the center to add the remaining ingredients

- Stir to combine

- Heat a 12-inch skillet and lightly grease it

- Spoon out pancakes using 1/3 cup measuring cup

- Cook until done and flip the pancake once only

NUTRITIONAL INFORMATION (per serving)

- Calories – 223

- Carbohydrate – 35g

- Protein – 7g

- Sodium – 196mg

- Potassium – 128mg

- Phosphorus – 100mg

- Dietary fiber – 2g

- Fat – 6g

Day #3: Vegetable Omelet

Omelet is a great breakfast option, and it's suitable for people who are not on dialysis. This omelet recipe is low in sodium, potassium, and phosphorus.

COOKING TIME: 5-10 MINUTES

INGREDIENTS FOR 1 SERVING

- Eggs – 2

- Water – 2tbsp

- Unsalted butter – 1tbsp

- Filling (seafood, meat, vegetables low in potassium/phosphorus) – ½ cup (so how to understand about nutritional info? With which filling or maybe without?)

METHOD

- Combine eggs and water

- Heat butter in a pan and pour in egg mixture

- Carefully tilt the pan when necessary a few times to let the mixture set evenly

- Fill the omelet with the filling of your choice (put the filling on the left or right side)

- Fold the omelet in half

- Serve

NUTRITIONAL INFORMATION (per serving)

- Calories – 255

- Carbohydrate – 1.3g

- Protein – 13g

- Sodium – 145mg

- Potassium – 122mg

- Phosphorus – 195mg

- Dietary fiber – 2g

- Fat – 20.3g

Day #4: Spicy Tofu Scrambler

You're a vegetarian or vegan and have kidney disease? This plant-based breakfast recipe will keep you full for hours and increase your energy levels.

COOKING TIME: 20 MINUTES

**INGREDIENTS FOR 2
SERVINGS**

SERVING SIZE: ½ cup

- Olive oil – 1tsp

- Red bell pepper (chopped) – ¼ cup

- Green bell pepper (chopped) – ¼ cup

- Firm tofu (less than 10% calcium) – 1 cup

- Onion powder – 1tsp

- Garlic powder – ¼ tsp

- Garlic (minced) – 1 clove

- Turmeric – 1/8tsp

METHOD

- Sauté garlic, bell peppers, and olive oil in a skillet

- Drain and rinse tofu and crumble it into the pan, then add other ingredients

- Cook on low to medium heat for about 20 minutes or until tofu turns golden brown

- Don't worry about water, and it will evaporate

NUTRITIONAL INFORMATION (per serving)

- Calories – 213

- Carbohydrate – 10g

- Protein – 18g

- Sodium – 24mg

- Potassium – 467mg

- Phosphorus – 242mg

- Dietary fiber – 2g

- Fat – 13g

Day #5: Homemade Sausage Patties

Just because you have a renal disease, it doesn't mean you are unable to enjoy sausage patties anymore. This kidney-friendly recipe is a wonderful breakfast option; you should definitely try.

COOKING TIME: 20 MINUTES

INGREDIENTS FOR 16 SERVINGS

SERVING SIZE: 1 patty

- Onion (chopped) – ½ cup

- Olive oil – 2tbsp

- Dried sage – 2tsp

- Black pepper – 1tsp

- Brown sugar – 1tbsp

- Red pepper flakes (crushed) – 1/8tsp

- Ground cloves – 1 pinch

- Fresh thyme (chopped) – 1tsp

- Egg yolk – 1

- Ground lean pork/beef – 2lbs/0.9kg

METHOD

- Over moderately low heat cook onion in olive oil for 8 to 10 minutes or until it softens and turns brown or golden

- Combine sage, pepper, cloves, sugar, and thyme in a small bowl

- In a separate bowl combine egg yolk, meat, and onion followed by mixed spices

- Mix thoroughly

- Make patties and fry them in a skillet over medium-high heat for 5 minutes per side

NUTRITIONAL INFORMATION (per serving)

- Calories – 173.3

- Carbohydrate – 1.5g

- Protein – 9.8g

- Sodium – 32.5mg

- Potassium – 270mg

- Phosphorus – 277mg

- Dietary fiber – 0.1g

- Fat – 14g

Day #6: Onion Bagel

For those times when you're in a hurry, onion bagel is a perfect breakfast option. This recipe contains tomato, but don't let it alarm you as only two slices are needed.

COOKING TIME: 2 MINUTES

INGREDIENTS FOR 2
SERVINGS

SERVING SIZE: ½ half of the bagel

- 2-oz bagel – 1

- Cream cheese – 2tbsp

- Tomato slices – 2

- Red onion slices – 2

- Low-sodium lemon pepper seasoning – 1tsp

METHOD

- Slice bagel in half and toast until it turns golden brown

- Over each bagel half spread cream cheese followed by onion and tomato slices, sprinkle with low-sodium lemon pepper seasoning

NUTRITIONAL INFORMATION (per serving)

- Calories – 134

- Carbohydrate – 19g

- Protein – 5g

- Sodium – 219mg

- Potassium – 162mg

- Phosphorus – 50mg

- Dietary fiber – 1.6g

- Fat – 6g

Day #7: Egg Muffins

Egg muffins are easy to make and are ideal for eating on the go. Of course, due to egg content, this recipe is not for dialysis patients.

COOKING TIME: 34 MINUTES

**INGREDIENTS FOR 8
SERVINGS**

SERVING SIZE: 1 muffin

- Bell peppers – 1 cup

- Onion – 1 cup

- Ground pork or beef – ½ lb/0.2kg

- Poultry seasoning – ¼ tsp

- Garlic powder – ¼ tsp

- Onion powder – ¼ tsp

- Herb seasoning blend – ½ tsp

- Eggs – 8

- Milk substitute – 2tbsp

- Salt (optional) – ¼ tsp

METHOD

- Preheat the oven to 350°F (176°C) and use a cooking spray to grease a muffin tin

- Dice onion and bell peppers

- Combine meat, poultry seasoning, garlic and onion powders, and seasoning in a bowl to create a sausage

- Cook sausage crumbles in a skillet for 12 minutes until they are done

- Mix eggs and milk substitute and combine with sausage crumbles and veggies

- Pour the mixture in the muffin tin and bake 18 to 22 minutes

NUTRITIONAL INFORMATION (per serving)

- Calories – 154

- Carbohydrate – 3g

- Protein – 12g

- Sodium – 155mg

- Potassium – 200mg

- Phosphorus – 154mg

- Dietary fiber – 0.5g

- Fat – 10g

Day #8: Sudden Quiche

What people love about quiches is their simplicity, but besides deliciousness, they can also be healthy. This quiche can also serve as a tasty dinner.

COOKING TIME: 45-60 MINUTES

INGREDIENTS FOR 6 SERVINGS

SERVING SIZE: 2 slices

- Eggs – 6

- Milk (2% or lower) – 1 cup

- Filling (leftover meat or vegetables) – 2 cups

- 9-inch deep-dish frozen pie shell – 1

- Grated cheese – 4oz (or 2oz if phosphorus is elevated)

METHOD

- Start by preheating the oven to 350°F (176°C)

- Combine milk, eggs, cheese, and filling of your choice

- Pour ingredients into a frozen pie shell and bake for 45 or 60 minutes or until a knife comes out clean when you insert it

- Let cool for 5 minutes before serving

NUTRITIONAL INFORMATION (per serving)

- Calories – 356

- Carbohydrate – 24g

- Protein – 16g

- Sodium – 409mg

- Potassium – 257mg

- Phosphorus – 278mg

- Dietary fiber – 22g

- Fat – 17.9g

Day #9: Loaded Veggie Eggs

Loaded veggie eggs recipe is super easy to follow, and it's needless to mention how delicious it is. To some people, it may seem odd that spinach is in the recipe, but it's important to mention you need to add fresh, not cooked spinach. Spinach becomes concentrated when it cooks, so using fresh alternative from time to time can be tolerated if you don't have serious kidney disease or are not on dialysis.

COOKING TIME: 7 MINUTES

INGREDIENTS FOR 2 SERVINGS

SERVING SIZE: ½ recipe

- Eggs – 4

- Cauliflower – 1 cup

- Fresh spinach – 3 cups

- Garlic (minced) – 1 clove

- Bell pepper (chopped) – ¼ cup

- Onion (chopped) – ¼ cup

- Black pepper – ¼ tsp

- Oil – 1tbsp

- Spring onion or fresh parsley

METHOD

- Combine eggs with black pepper and set aside

- Heat oil in a skillet and add bell pepper and onion that you will sauté until they are golden and translucent, then add garlic, cauliflower, and spinach

- Turn heat to medium-low and cover the skillet, cook for 5 minutes

- Add eggs to the skillet and stir

- Once eggs are cooked, sprinkle them with parsley or spring onion

NUTRITIONAL INFORMATION (per serving)

- Calories – 240

- Carbohydrate – 7.8g

- Protein – 15.3g

- Sodium – 195mg

- Potassium – 605.2mg

- Phosphorus – 253.6mg

- Dietary fiber – 2.7g

- Fat – 16.6g

Day #10: Fast Burritos

Burrito is always a great choice, so you may start your day with it as well. The reason is simple; it will fill you up, so you'll consume a lower amount of calories during the day and thereby lower intake of potassium and phosphorus as well as sodium.

COOKING TIME: 10 MINUTES

**INGREDIENTS FOR 4
SERVINGS**

SERVING SIZE: 1 burrito

- Olive oil – 1 ½ tsp

- Red bell pepper (diced) – ½

- Scallions (sliced) – 4

- Eggs (beaten) – 8

- Corn tortillas - 4

METHOD

- Heat oil over medium heat and add bell pepper and green onion. Cook for 3 minutes or until softened

- Add eggs to the vegetables and cook for 5 minutes or until eggs are done

- Microwave tortillas for 2 minutes

- Add egg mixture into warm tortillas, roll them up and eat

NUTRITIONAL INFORMATION (per serving)

- Calories – 232

- Carbohydrate – 16g

- Protein – 14g

- Sodium – 152mg

- Potassium – 211mg

- Phosphorus – 207mg

- Dietary fiber – 6g

- Fat – 11.3g

Day #11: Easy and Simple Crepe

In the mood for crepes? It's time to make them. Don't worry; you can do it without too much hassle and unnecessary complications.

COOKING TIME: 60 MINUTES

INGREDIENTS FOR 16 SERVINGS

SERVING SIZE: 1 crepe

- Eggs – 3

- Milk or milk substitute – 1 – 1/3 cups

- All-purpose white flour – ¾ cup

- Butter (melted) – 3tbsp

METHOD

- Mix eggs and milk and combine with flour, cover and let the mixture sit for 1 hour

- Pour batter into the bowl and add butter

- Heat skillet over medium-high heat and coat with a cooking spray

- Pour batter into the pan, move the pan when necessary to make the crepes even until they turn golden brown

- Combine crepe with sidings of your choice

NUTRITIONAL INFORMATION (per serving)

- Calories – 63

- Carbohydrate – 6g

- Protein – 3g

- Sodium – 29mg

- Potassium – 50mg

- Phosphorus – 45mg

- Dietary fiber – 0.1g

- Fat – 3g

Day #12: Corn Idlis

Corn idlis is a simple Indian meal that will awaken your taste buds. What you'll love about this breakfast snack is its simplicity. You can prepare it easily and without too much hassle. Corn idli is satiating, meaning you won't be hungry for hours.

COOKING TIME: 20 MINUTES

INGREDIENTS FOR 4 SERVINGS

SERVING SIZE: 3 idlis

- Vegetable oil – 2tbsp

- Mustard seeds – 1tsp

- Semolina – ¼ cup

- Green chilies (chopped) – 2

- Salt – 1/8tsp

- Yogurt – ¼ cup

- Water – ¼ cup

- Corn (grated) – ¼ cup

- Paneer cheese – ¼ cup

- Cilantro (chopped) – 1tbsp

- Coriander (chopped) – 1tbsp

- Ghee – 1tbsp

METHOD

- Heat vegetable oil in a saucepan and add mustard seeds

- When seeds splutter proceed to add semolina, salt, and chilies, and roast them until semolina turns brownish

- Remove pan from the stove

- Combine yogurt and water and add together with corn, cheese, and cilantro to semolina mixture, stir thoroughly and let sit for 10 minutes

- Use ghee to grease idli mold and add small portions of the batter

- Steam and cook idli for 10 minutes sprinkle with cilantro and coriander

NUTRITIONAL INFORMATION (per serving)

- Calories – 175

- Carbohydrate – 14g

- Protein – 5g

- Sodium – 214mg

- Potassium – 140mg

- Phosphorus – 89mg

- Dietary fiber – 0.8g

- Fat – 11g

Day #13: Plain Egg Whites

Egg whites are an excellent breakfast choice for people with kidney disease who are not on dialysis. Plain, healthy, and simple – the winning combination.

COOKING TIME: 5 MINUTES

**INGREDIENTS FOR 1
SERVING**

SERVING SIZE: 1 cup

- Egg whites – 8oz/220gr

- Oil – 1tsp

METHOD

- Pour egg whites into a greased pan and cook over medium heat until done

- Sprinkle low-sodium herbal seasonings to enhance the taste, if you'd prefer

NUTRITIONAL INFORMATION (per serving)

- Calories – 165

- Carbohydrate – 2g

- Protein – 28g

- Sodium – 428mg

- Potassium – 420mg

- Phosphorus – 39mg

- Dietary fiber – 0g

- Fat – 5g

Day #14: Baked Pancakes

Let's add an interesting twist to "regular" pancakes. Baked pancakes are easier to make and quite versatile as you can add any type of spread you want.

COOKING TIME: 25 MINUTES

> **INGREDIENTS FOR 4 SERVINGS**

SERVING SIZE: 1 wedge

- Eggs – 2

- Milk or milk substitute – ½ cup

- All-purpose white flour – ½ cup

- Salt – ¼ tsp

- Nutmeg – 1/8 tsp

- Oil – 1tbsp

METHOD

- Preheat the oven to 450°F (232°C)

- Combine eggs and milk in a bowl and add salt, flour, and nutmeg

- Pour oil in an ovenproof skillet and place in the oven for 5 minutes

- Pour pancake batter into the pan, place it into the oven, and bake for 18 to 20 minutes

- Slice into wedges and eat with favorite syrup or spread

NUTRITIONAL INFORMATION (per serving)

- Calories – 189

- Carbohydrate – 27g

- Protein – 8g

- Sodium – 206mg

- Potassium – 157mg

- Phosphorus – 135mg

- Dietary fiber – 0.9g

- Fat – 5g

BONUS: Baked Egg Cups

Eggs are versatile and allow us to combine them with a wide range of ingredients or prepare them in many ways. Have you ever baked eggs? Now you have the chance to do so. Make this breakfast when you have leftover of white rice.

COOKING TIME: 15 MINUTES

INGREDIENTS FOR 12 SERVINGS

SERVING SIZE: 1 egg cup

- Rice (cooked) – 3 cups

- Cheddar cheese (shredded) – 4oz/110rg

- Green chilies (diced) – 4oz/110gr

- Pimentos (diced, drained) – 2oz/60gr

- Skim milk – ½ cup

- Eggs (beaten) – 2

- Black pepper – ½ tsp

- Ground cumin – ½ tsp

METHOD

- Combine all two ounces of cheese with other ingredients into a bowl

- Coat muffin tin with cooking spray

- Add the mixture into 12 muffin cups and sprinkle with the remainder of cheese

- Bake for 15 minutes or until the mixture is set over 400°F (204°C)

NUTRITIONAL INFORMATION (per serving)

- Calories – 109

- Carbohydrate – 13g

- Protein – 5g

- Sodium – 79mg

- Potassium – 82mg

- Phosphorus – 91mg

- Dietary fiber – 0.5mg

- Fat – 4g

Chapter 6: Lunch

What's for lunch today? Sometimes no ideas come to mind despite our efforts to think of a nice, delicious, and healthy meal. With this book, you'll avoid those problems. Throughout this chapter, you will find easy-to-make and kidney-friendly lunch ideas.

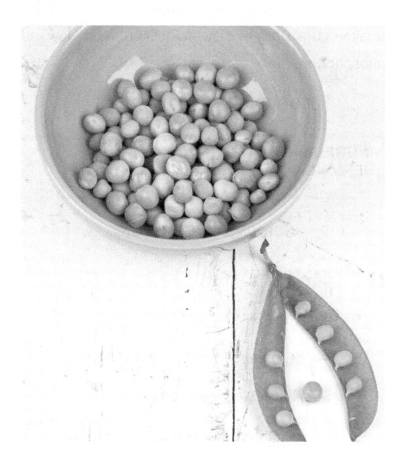

Day #1: Lemon Orzo Spring Salad

Here's a perfect dish you can make to maintain your weight and still feel full. You can make this salad all-year-round, especially in spring, when you can experiment with different ingredients and vegetables (make sure they're low-potassium and low in phosphorus).

COOKING TIME: 20 MINUTES

INGREDIENTS FOR 4 SERVING

SERVING SIZE: 1½ cups

- Orzo pasta – ¾ cup

- Red peppers (diced) – ¼ cup

- Yellow peppers (diced) – ¼ cup

- Green peppers (diced) – ¼ cup

- Red onion (diced) – ½ cup

- Zucchini (cubed) – 2 cups

- Olive oil – ¼ cup and 2tbsp

- Lemon juice – 3tbsp

- Lemon zest – 1tsp

- Parmesan cheese (grated) – 3tbsp

- Rosemary (chopped) – 2tbsp

- Black pepper – ½ tsp

- Oregano – ½ tsp

- Red pepper flakes – ½ tsp

METHOD

- Cook orzo pasta according to the instructions on the packaging, about 10 minutes, and set aside

- Over medium-high heat sauté two tablespoons of oil with peppers, onions, and zucchini until they become translucent

- In a bowl combine lemon zest, lemon juice, ¼ cup of olive oil, pepper, rosemary, oregano, and red pepper flakes then add pasta and vegetables, stir thoroughly and sprinkle grated parmesan cheese over the salad

NUTRITIONAL INFORMATION (per serving)

- Calories – 330

- Carbohydrate – 28g

- Protein – 6g

- Sodium – 79mg

- Potassium – 376mg

- Phosphorus – 134mg

- Dietary fiber – 5g

- Fat – 22g

Day #2: Chicken and Orang Salad Sandwich

The sandwich is not just a snack or quick meal you eat at work. You can turn it into a delicious lunch that also happens to be low in protein, potassium, phosphorus, and sodium.

COOKING TIME: 5 MINUTES

> **INGREDIENTS FOR 6 SERVINGS**

SERVING SIZE: ½ cup

- Cooked chicken (chopped) – 1 cup

- Celery (diced) – ½ cup

- Green pepper (chopped) – ½ cup

- Onion (sliced) – ¼ cup

- Mandarin orange – 1 cup

- Mayonnaise – 1/3 cup

METHOD

- Combine chicken, pepper, onion, and celery in a bowl and mix thoroughly

- Add mayonnaise and mandarin oranges

- Make a sandwich or serve on a bread

NUTRITIONAL INFORMATION (per serving)

- Calories – 170

- Carbohydrate – 6g

- Protein – 12g

- Sodium – 97mg

- Potassium – 241mg

- Phosphorus – 106mg

- Dietary fiber – 0.7g

- Fat – 5.1g

Day #3: Herb-Roasted Chicken Breast

Chicken breast is a wonderful addition to any meal, or it can be served on its own. This time for lunch makes sure you use the power of herbs to introduce a variety of flavors to your palate.

COOKING TIME: 25 MINUTES

INGREDIENTS FOR 4 SERVINGS

SERVING SIZE: 4 oz

- Chicken breasts (boneless, skinless) – 1lb/0.45kg

- Onion – 1

- Garlic – 1-2 cloves

- Herb seasoning blend – 2tbsp

- Ground black pepper – 1tsp

- Olive oil – ¼ cup

METHOD

- Marinate chicken breasts in onion, garlic, seasoning, pepper, and olive oil mixture for 4 hours or overnight

- Preheat the oven to 350°F (176°C)

- Cover the baking dish with foil, arrange chicken breasts and cover with marinade

- Bake for 20 minutes and broil 5 minutes

- Serve hot

NUTRITIONAL INFORMATION (per serving)

- Calories – 270

- Carbohydrate – 3g

- Protein – 26g

- Sodium – 53mg

- Potassium – 491mg

- Phosphorus – 252mg

- Dietary fiber – 0.6g

- Fat – 17g

Day #4: Low-Sodium Chicken Soup

Chicken soup helps us feel better when we're sick, but it's also a delicious meal for lunch or dinner. Most recipes for chicken soup are high in sodium, but this one is different, and it's safe for patients with kidney disease.

COOKING TIME: 75 MINUTES

INGREDIENTS FOR 10 SERVINGS

. SERVING SIZE: 1½ cups

- Chicken breast (cooked, boneless, skinless) – 1lb/0.45kg

- Onion – 1tbsp

- Celery – 4 stalks

- Parsley – 2tbsp

- Carrots – 1 cup

- Butter – 1tbsp

- Water – 7 ½ cups

- Chicken broth (low-sodium) – 5 cups

- Black pepper – 1/8 tsp

- Frozen mixed vegetables – 1 cup

METHOD

- Cut chicken into dices and set aside

- Sauté butter and onion in a 4-quart pot until tender or 5 minutes

- Pour chicken brother and water to a pot, bring to a boil

- Add chicken, pepper, parsley, celery to a pot and simmer for 30 minutes

- Add carrots to remaining ingredients and simmer for 20 minutes, add frozen vegetables and let simmer for additional 20 minutes

NUTRITIONAL INFORMATION (per serving)

- Calories – 97

- Carbohydrate – 5g

- Protein – 13g

- Sodium – 301mg

- Potassium – 274mg

- Phosphorus – 116mg

- Dietary fiber – 1.6g

- Fat – 3g

Day #5: Grilled Peppers and Onions

Bell peppers are beneficial for people with kidney disease, as well as onions. Not only are they good for your health, but they are also colorful and easy on the eye.

COOKING TIME: 18 MINUTES

INGREDIENTS FOR 4 SERVINGS

SERVING SIZE: 1 skewer

- Red onion – 1

- Vidalia onion – 1

- Red bell pepper – 1

- Yellow bell pepper – 1

- Green bell pepper – 1

- Olive oil – 1/3 cup

- Salt – ¼ tsp

- Black pepper – ¾ tsp

METHOD

- Seed bell peppers and slice them, quarter-cut onions

- Combine all ingredients in a large bowl

- Arrange vegetables on skewers and grill for 18 minutes

NUTRITIONAL INFORMATION (per serving)

- Calories – 154

- Carbohydrate – 11g

- Protein – 1g

- Sodium – 146mg

- Potassium – 244mg

- Phosphorus – 41mg

- Dietary fiber – 1.7g

- Fat – 13g

Day #6: Crunchy Quinoa Salad

Crunchy quinoa salad combines a plethora of healthy and delicious ingredients for a satiating lunch. Though this recipe contains tomatoes in such doses they will not impact too much on your disease.

COOKING TIME: 15 MINUTES

INGREDIENTS FOR 8 SERVINGS

SERVING SIZE: ½ cup

- Quinoa (rinsed) – 1 cup

- Water – 2 cups

- Cherry tomatoes (diced) – 5

- Cucumber (diced) – ½ cup

- Green onions (chopped) – 3

- Mint (chopped) – ¼ cup

- Parsley (chopped) – ½ cup

- Lemon juice – 2tbsp

- Lemon zest – 1tbsp

- Olive oil – 4tbsp

- Parmesan cheese (grated) – ¼ cup

- Lettuce (separated into cups) – ½ head

METHOD

- Rinse quinoa and drain well before you place it in a pan and toast for 2 minutes over medium-high heat

- Pour 2 cups of water and bring to a boil, then reduce the heat to low and let simmer for 8 to 10 minutes

- Fluff using a fork

- In a separate bowl combine cucumbers, tomato, onions, herbs, and lemon juice and zest with olive oil, and add quinoa mixture to them

- Using a spoon place quinoa mixture into lettuce leaves and garnish with cheese

NUTRITIONAL INFORMATION (per serving)

- Calories – 158

- Carbohydrate – 16g

- Protein – 5g

- Sodium – 46mg

- Potassium – 237mg

- Phosphorus – 129mg

- Dietary fiber – 2.3g

- Fat – 9g

Day #7: Savory Salmon Dip

Salmon is abundant in Omega-3 fatty acids, which are essential for your health. This dip requires a few easy steps, and you can serve it on its own, with celery and other vegetables, or as a side dish to some other meal. Options are endless.

COOKING TIME: 66 MINUTES

> **INGREDIENTS FOR 12 SERVINGS**

SERVING SIZE: ¼ cup

- Salmon (skinless, boneless) – 1lb/0.45kg

- Smoked paprika – 2tsp

- Cream cheese – 1 cup

- Capers – ¼ cup

- Lemon juice – ¼ cup

- Lemon zest – 1tsp

- Red onions (diced) – 2tbsp

- Ground black pepper – 1tsp

91

- Parsley (chopped) – 1tbsp.

- Water – 2 cups

METHOD

- Over medium-high heat poach salmon with 1tsp of smoked paprika and 2 cups of water for 4 to 6 minutes

- Remove from the heat and let sit for 30 minutes

- Combine other ingredients

- Add salmon to the bowl with other ingredients and chill for 20 to 30 minutes before serving

NUTRITIONAL INFORMATION (per serving)

- Calories – 133

- Carbohydrate – 2g

- Protein – 10g

- Sodium – 147mg

- Potassium – 259mg

- Phosphorus – 110mg

- Dietary fiber – 0mg

- Fat – 9g

Day #8: Beef Stew with Mushrooms and Carrots

Stew is a hearty meal and the perfect lunch idea for cold or winter days. This particular stew combines mushrooms, beef, and a plethora of herbs and other ingredients that not only taste great but have a wonderful scent too.

COOKING TIME: 2 HOURS

**INGREDIENTS FOR 8
SERVINGS**

SERVING SIZE:1 cup

- White potato – 1 cup

- Olive oil – 2tbsp (divided)

- Shiitake mushrooms (sliced) – 1 cup

- Onion – 2 cups

- Garlic – 3 cloves

- Dry red wine – 1 cup

- White flour – 1/3 cup

94

- Lean beef – 2lbs

- Herb seasoning – ¾ tsp

- Beef broth (low-sodium) – 4 cups

- Thyme – ½ tbsp

- Bay leaf – 1

- Carrot – 2 cups

- Black pepper – ½ tsp

METHOD

- Peel and cube potato, and double-boil or soak to reduce potassium levels

- Heat 2tsp of olive oil in a Dutch oven over medium-high heat and add onion which you will cook until it becomes tender or 5 minutes. Then, add mushrooms, thyme, and cook for more 5 minutes

- Add garlic and cook for 1 minute

- Pour red wine to the mixture and stir

- Start coating beef in flour

- Heat 2tsp of olive oil in a large frying pan over medium heat, add half of beef and season with seasoning blend

- Cook beef until it browns on all sides. Repeat the same process with the remainder of the meat

- Add beef to the mushroom mixture followed by broth, bay leaf, thyme, and bring to a boil

- Decrease the heat to medium-low and let simmer for 1 hour

- Drain potatoes and add them along with carrot to a pot with beef and mushrooms, let simmer for 1 hour uncovered

- Discard bay leaf, add black pepper and herbal seasoning

NUTRITIONAL INFORMATION (per serving)

- Calories – 282

- Carbohydrate – 15g

- Protein – 33g

- Sodium – 110mg

- Potassium – 534mg

- Phosphorus – 252mg

- Dietary fiber – 2.5g

- Fat – 10g

y #9: Mediterranean Green Beans

Mediterranean diet is considered to be the healthiest diet in the world. So, we can borrow their ingredients to make a delicious and healthy lunch, such as this green beans recipe.

COOKING TIME: 5 MINUTES

INGREDIENTS FOR 4 SERVINGS

SERVING SIZE:1 cup

- Green beans (cut into small pieces) – 1lb/0.45kg

- Water – ¾ cup

- Olive oil – 2 ½ tsp

- Garlic (minced) – 3 cloves

- Lemon juice – 3tbsp

- Ground black pepper – 1/8 tsp

METHOD

- In a large skillet bring water to a boil, add beans and cook for 3 minutes, then drain them and set aside

- Sauté garlic and beans in a skillet for 1 minute over medium-high heat

- Add pepper and juice then sauté for an additional minute

NUTRITIONAL INFORMATION (per serving)

- Calories – 71

- Carbohydrate – 10g

- Protein – 2g

- Sodium – 2g

- Potassium – 186mg

- Phosphorus – 37mg

- Dietary fiber – 3.7g

- Fat – 3g

Day #10: Turkey Waldorf Salad

This unique salad combines apples and turkey with outstanding results. Fast to make and delicious to eat, the perfect lunch solution.

COOKING TIME: 5 MINUTES

INGREDIENTS FOR 6 SERVINGS

SERVING SIZE: ½ cup

- Turkey breast (cooked/boiled) – 12oz/340gr

- Red apples – 3

- Celery – 1 cup

- Onion – ½ cup

- Mayonnaise – ¼ cup

- Apple juice – 2tbsp

METHOD

- Cut turkey in small cubes and dice apples, onion, and celery

- Combine all ingredients in a bowl, stir well

- Chill before serving

NUTRITIONAL INFORMATION (per serving)

- Calories – 200

- Carbohydrate – 8g

- Protein – 17g

- Sodium – 128mg

- Potassium – 296mg

- Phosphorus – 136mg

- Dietary fiber – 1.9g

- Fat – 11g

Day #11: Spring Vegetable Soup

This spring vegetable soup is rich in nutrients and unbelievably delicious. Yet, it takes only a few simple steps to prepare it.

COOKING TIME: 60 MINUTES

INGREDIENTS FOR 5 SERVINGS

SERVING SIZE: 1 cup

- Green beans – 1 cup

- Celery – ¾ cup

- Onion – ½ cup

- Carrot – ½ cup

- Mushroom – ½ cup

- Frozen corn – ½ cup

- Roma tomato – 1

- Olive oil – 2tbsp

- Frozen corn – ½ cup

- Vegetable broth (low-sodium) – 4 cups

- Oregano – 1tsp

- Garlic powder – 1tsp

- Salt – ¼ tsp

METHOD

- Cut beans, celery, onion, mushrooms, carrot, and tomato in small pieces

- Sauté celery and onion in olive oil until they are tender, then add remaining ingredients into the pot and bring to a boil.

- Decrease the heat and simmer for 45 to 60 minutes

NUTRITIONAL INFORMATION (per serving)

- Calories – 114

- Carbohydrate – 13g

- Protein – 2g

- Sodium – 262mg

- Potassium – 400mg

- Phosphorus – 108mg

- Dietary fiber – 3.4g

- Fat – 6g

Day #12: Egg Fried Rice

The Asian-inspired dish is perfect for people who don't have much time, and they have some leftovers in the fridge. Eggs, rice, vegetables – a rhapsody of tastes on the plate.

COOKING TIME: 10 MINUTES

INGREDIENTS FOR 10 SERVINGS

SERVING SIZE: ½ cup

- Dark sesame oil – 2tsp

- Eggs – 2

- Egg whites – 2

- Canola oil – 1tbsp

- Bean sprouts – 1 cup

- Green onions (chopped) – 1/3 cup

- Rice (cooked, cold) – 4 cups

- Peas (frozen, thawed) – 1 cup

- Ground black pepper – ¼ tsp

METHOD

- In a small bowl combine sesame oil, eggs and egg whites, set aside

- Over medium-high heat stir-fry egg mixture until it's done then add bean sprouts and onions, stir-fry for an additional 2 minutes

- Add peas and rice into the mixture and fry until it is heated evenly

- Season with pepper

NUTRITIONAL INFORMATION (per serving)

- Calories – 137

- Carbohydrate – 21g

- Protein – 5g

- Sodium – 38mg

- Potassium – 89mg

- Phosphorus – 67mg

- Dietary fiber – 1.3g

- Fat – 4g

Day #13: Creamy Cauliflower

If you're a fan of mashed potatoes, here's a great alternative that won't get potassium levels through the roof. Creamy cauliflower turns out to be a filling lunch that you can serve on its own or accompanied by chicken or other quality protein sources.

COOKING TIME: 35 MINUTES

INGREDIENTS FOR 6 SERVINGS

SERVING SIZE: ½ cup

- Cauliflower – 8 cups

- Water – 5-6 cups or enough to cover florets

- Garlic – 1tsp

- Leek bulb – 1

- Salt – ¼ tsp

- White pepper – 1/8 tsp

- Unsalted butter – 1tbsp

107

METHOD

- Break the cauliflower into florets, place them in the pot and pour water over it

- Bring water to a boil and cook for 20 minutes, drain water making sure there's 1 cup left with cauliflower, then add leeks and garlic

- Cook for 10 to 15 minutes or until cauliflower and leeks are tender, then drain

- Blend vegetables into a mashed potato-like mixture

- Stir in the butter and season with salt and pepper

NUTRITIONAL INFORMATION (per serving)

- Calories – 64

- Carbohydrate – 9g

- Protein – 3g

- Sodium – 116mg

- Potassium – 256mg

- Phosphorus – 58mg

- Dietary fiber – 4.8mg

- Fat – 3g

Day #14: Pasta Primavera

Pasta is a quick and easy lunch solution for those times when you're in a hurry, expecting guests, and want to make something that everyone likes. This recipe shows you can make pasta with a healthy twist.

COOKING TIME: 20 MINUTES

INGREDIENTS FOR 6 SERVINGS

SERVING SIZE:1-3/4 cup

- Pasta (uncooked) – 12oz/340gr

- Water – 4qt

- Frozen vegetables – 12oz/340gr

- Chicken broth (low-sodium) – 14oz/400gr

- Half and half creamer – ¼ cup

- Flour – 2tbsp

- Garlic powder – ¼ tsp

- Parmesan cheese (grated) – ¼ cup

METHOD

- In separate pots cook pasta (in four quarts of water) and for about 10 minutes or until done, omit the salt, then drain

- Heat chicken broth in a stockpot over low heat and add flour, whisk thoroughly to avoid clumps

- Add garlic powder and a half and half, stir thoroughly, let simmer for 5 to 10 minutes

- Add vegetables and pasta to chicken broth ingredients

- Before serving sprinkle with parmesan

NUTRITIONAL INFORMATION (per serving)

- Calories – 273

- Carbohydrate – 48g

- Protein – 13g

- Sodium – 115mg

- Potassium – 251mg

- Phosphorus – 154mg

- Dietary fiber – 4.5g

- Fat – 3g

BONUS: Cucumber Salad

Cucumber salad is crispy, refreshing, and low in calories. It's ideal for weight management, which is also important for people with kidney disease.

COOKING TIME: 3 MINUTES

INGREDIENTS FOR 4 SERVINGS

SERVING SIZE: ½ cup

- Cucumber (sliced) – 2 cups

- Caesar salad or Italian salad dressing – 2tbsp

- Ground black pepper to taste

METHOD

- Combine cucumber slices and salad dressing in a bowl with a lid

- Shake the bowl

- Sprinkle with pepper before putting the salad into the fridge

NUTRITIONAL INFORMATION (per serving)

- Calories – 27

- Carbohydrate – 3g

- Protein – 0g

- Sodium – 74mg

- Potassium – 90mg

- Phosphorus – 14mg

- Dietary fiber – 0g

- Fat – 2g

Chapter 7: Dinner

The most common reason why some people fail to adhere to a healthy diet is that they think it would be impossible to have a delicious yet healthy dinner. When you come home from work, all you want is to eat something tasty, that doesn't take ages to prepare, and you want to use some everyday ingredients. You'll be happy to know that the renal diet checks all those boxes easily. This chapter is reserved for kidney-friendly dinner.

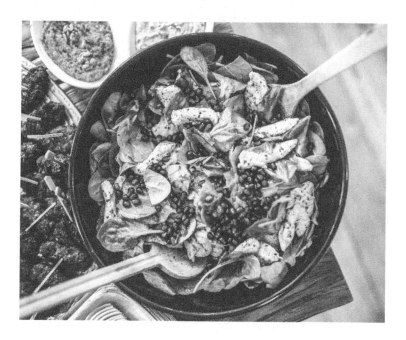

Day #1: Chicken or Beef Enchiladas

Enchiladas are a great dinner choice for the whole family. The best thing about this recipe is that it doesn't require too many ingredients, and you can prepare it even when you're tired after work.

COOKING TIME: 20 MINUTES

INGREDIENTS FOR 6
SERVINGS

SERVING SIZE: 1 enchilada

- Ground chicken or beef – 1lb/0.45kg

- Onion (chopped) – ½ cup

- Cumin – 1tsp

- Black pepper – ½ tsp

- Garlic (chopped) – 1 clove

- Corn tortillas – 12

- Enchilada sauce (low sodium) – 1 can

METHOD

- First, preheat oven to 375°F (190°C)

- In frying pan brown the meat of your choice and add garlic, onion, pepper, and cumin, stir thoroughly until onions soften

- Fry tortillas in a separate pan and dip each into enchilada sauce

- Fill tortilla with the meat mixture and roll it up

- Bake until enchiladas are golden brown, or you may sprinkle them with cheese and bake until it melts

NUTRITIONAL INFORMATION (per serving)

- Calories – 235

- Carbohydrate – 30

- Protein – 13g

- Sodium – 201mg

- Potassium – 222mg

- Phosphorus – 146mg

- Dietary fiber – 14g

- Fat – 6.9g

Day #2: Mediterranean Pizza

Pizza lovers rejoice! This popular Italian meal doesn't necessarily have to be unhealthy when you choose all the right ingredients. Mediterranean pizza is delicious and colorful, the ideal treat for dinner.

COOKING TIME: 15 MINUTES

INGREDIENTS FOR 12 SERVINGS

SERVING SIZE: 1 slice

- Crust – 1

- Olive oil – 1tbsp

- Garlic (sliced) – 2 cloves

- Roma tomato (sliced) – 1

- Basil (sliced) – 10 leaves

- Ricotta or goat cheese – 3oz

METHOD

- Preheat the oven to 450°F(232°C) and drizzle pizza crust with olive oil

119

- Place garlic evenly across the crust and cover it with tomato slices

- Use basil to sprinkle and decorate pizza and add cheese on top

- Bake for 10 to 15 minutes

NUTRITIONAL INFORMATION (per serving)

- Calories – 176

- Carbohydrate – 18g

- Protein – 7g

- Sodium – 240mg

- Potassium – 86g

- Phosphorus – 90g

- Dietary fiber – 8g

- Fat – 0g

Day #3: Pancit Guisado

Pancit guisado is a Filipino noodle dish. It is prepared in everyday situations, but also in some special occasions. If you've never prepared this meal before, you can have it for dinner. It's easy!

COOKING TIME: 20 MINUTES

INGREDIENTS FOR 6 SERVINGS

SERVING SIZE: 1 ½ cup

- Rice stick noodles – 8oz/230gr

- Vegetable oil – ¼ cup

- Garlic (minced) – 3 cloves

- Onion (chopped) – ½

- Chicken breast (skinless) – 1lb/0,45kg

- Green cabbage (shredded) – 1 ½ cups

- Carrot – 1

- Soy sauce (reduced sodium) – 1tbsp

- Chicken broth (reduced sodium) – 1 cup

- Celery (sliced) – 1 stalk

- Green onions (chopped) – 2

- Lemon (optional) - 1

METHOD

- Soak noodles in warm water for 5 minutes, drain them and set aside

- Heat oil over medium heat in a pan and add onion and garlic, sauté them for 5 minutes

- Add cabbage, meat, and carrot to the pan and fry occasionally stirring for 3 minutes

- Add soy sauce, celery, and chicken broth, and let simmer for 3 minutes

- Add rice noodles to the mixture in the pan and simmer for additional 3 minutes

- Garnish with green onions and sprinkle with lemon juice when serving

NUTRITIONAL INFORMATION (per serving)

- Calories – 287

- Carbohydrate – 39g

- Protein – 19g

- Sodium – 194mg

- Potassium – 391mg

- Phosphorus – 183mg

- Dietary fiber – 2.8g

- Fat – 11.7g

Day #4: Zucchini Sauté

Here's a recipe that turns dinner into a delicious, yet healthy snack. This is ideal for those nights when you're not too hungry but still feel like eating something yummy.

COOKING TIME: 5-10 MINUTES

INGREDIENTS FOR 6 SERVINGS

SERVING SIZE: ½ cup

- Zucchini (sliced) – 3-4

- Milk or milk substitute – 1 cup

- Flour – ½ cup

- Parmesan cheese (grated) – ¼ cup

- Thyme – ½ tsp

- Basil – ½ tsp

- Tarragon – ½ tsp

- Oil – 2tbsp

- Pepper to taste

METHOD

- Soak zucchini in milk while you combine flour, parmesan, pepper, and herbs in a bowl

- In a large skillet heat vegetable oil

- Dip zucchini in bowl mixture and sauté until done

- Serve hot

NUTRITIONAL INFORMATION (per serving)

- Calories – 121

- Carbohydrate – 13g

- Protein – 4g

- Sodium – 75mg

- Potassium – 374mg

- Phosphorus – 91mg

- Dietary fiber – 1.5g

- Fat – 6g

Day #5: Creamy Tuna

Tuna and pasta are a winning combination, and you can indulge in this delicious meal on a renal diet, too. Add mayonnaise and vegetables to take this meal to a whole new level.

COOKING TIME: 10-20 MINUTES

INGREDIENTS FOR 4 SERVINGS

SERVING SIZE: 1 cup

- Mayonnaise – ¾ cup

- Vinegar – 2tbsp

- Shell macaroni (cooked) – 1 ½ cups

- Tuna (drained) – 1 can (water-packed or unsalted)

- Peas (cooked) – ½ cup

- Celery (chopped) – ½ cup

- Dried dill – 1tbsp

126

METHOD

- Mix mayo, vinegar, and macaroni in a large bowl add other ingredients

- Cover and chill

NUTRITIONAL INFORMATION (per serving)

- Calories – 415

- Carbohydrate – 15g

- Protein – 12g

- Sodium – 258mg

- Potassium – 175mg

- Phosphorus – 116mg

- Dietary fiber – 2.2g

- Fat – 15.5g

Day #6: Red Cabbage Casserole

This is a healthier alternative to the casserole and the perfect meal for patients with kidney disease. Red cabbage casserole is going to awaken your taste buds, and it's also pretty on the plate.

COOKING TIME: 2 ½ HOURS

INGREDIENTS FOR 8 SERVINGS

SERVING SIZE: ½ cup

- Red cabbage (shredded) – 1

- Onion (chopped) – 1 cup

- Apples (peeled, sliced) – 3 cups

- Red wine vinegar – ¼ cup

- Water – ¼ cup

- Brown sugar – 2tbsp

- Black pepper – ¼ tsp

- Unsalted butter – 2tbsp

METHOD

- Preheat the oven to 300°F(148°C)

- In a large bowl combine all ingredients except butter

- Transfer ingredients to a casserole dish and dot with butter, cover the dish and cook for two and a half hours

NUTRITIONAL INFORMATION (per serving)

- Calories – 79

- Carbohydrate – 13g

- Protein – 1g

- Sodium – 13mg

- Potassium – 161mg

- Phosphorus – 23mg

- Dietary fiber – 2g

- Fat – 3g

ay #7: Hawaiian Chicken Salad Sandwich

Ideally, dinners should be light and feature a healthy snack or two. Hawaiian chicken sandwich checks that box easily, and it also brings the tastes of Hawaii wherever you are.

COOKING TIME: 5-10 MINUTES

> **INGREDIENTS FOR 4 SERVINGS**

SERVING SIZE: 1 cup chicken salad, 1 piece of tortilla/flatbread

- Chicken (cooked, diced) – 2 cups

- Pineapple tidbits – 1 cup

- Low-fat mayonnaise – ½ cup

- Green bell pepper – ½ cup

- Carrot – 1/3 cup

- Black pepper – ½ tsp

- Flatbread – 4 pieces

METHOD

- Dice and chop the ingredients

- Combine ingredients in a bowl and place in the fridge until you need them

- Serve chicken mixture on flatbread

NUTRITIONAL INFORMATION (per serving)

- Calories – 349

- Carbohydrate – 24g

- Protein – 22g

- Sodium – 398mg

- Potassium – 333mg

- Phosphorus – 167mg

- Dietary fiber – 1.5g

- Fat – 17g

Day #8: Italian Meatballs

Italian meatballs are absolutely delicious, whether they're on their own or in combination with other ingredients on the plate. Meat, spices, and herbs and less than five steps to follow lead you to the best meatballs you've ever tried.

COOKING TIME: 15 MINUTES

INGREDIENTS FOR 12 SERVINGS

SERVING SIZE: 2 meatballs

- Ground beef – 1.5lbs/0,7kg

- Eggs (beaten) – 2

- Dry oatmeal flakes – ½ cup

- Parmesan cheese – 3tbsp

- Olive oil – ½ tbsp

- Garlic powder – ½ tbsp

- Oregano – 1tsp

- Onion (chopped) – ½ cup

- Black pepper – ½ tsp

METHOD

- Preheat the oven to 375°F(190°C)

- Mix all ingredients in a bowl, make meatballs and place them on a baking sheet

- Bake for 10 to 15 minutes

NUTRITIONAL INFORMATION (per serving)

- Calories – 163

- Carbohydrate – 4g

- Protein – 13g

- Sodium – 72mg

- Potassium – 199mg

- Phosphorus – 125mg

- Dietary fiber – 0.2g

- Fat – 6.5g

#9: Green Bean Casserole

This is not your typical casserole. Green bean, crushed tortilla chips, spices, and crunchy breadcrumbs take the casserole game to a whole new level.

COOKING TIME: 15 MINUTES

INGREDIENTS FOR 6
SERVINGS

SERVING SIZE: 3 oz

- String green beans – 12oz/350gr

- Hot sauce – 2tbsp

- Cheddar or gorgonzola cheese – ¼ cup

- Butter (melted, unsalted) – 2tbsp

- Panko breadcrumbs – ½ cup

- Green onions (chopped) – 2tbsp

- Tortilla chips (unsalted, plain, crushed) – ½ cup

METHOD

- Preheat the oven to 375°F(190°C) and in the meantime cut string beans, combine them with hot sauce and pour into the casserole dish

- In a small bowl combine remaining ingredients, sprinkle them evenly over green bean mixture and bake for 12 to 15 minutes or until it reaches preferred level of crispiness

NUTRITIONAL INFORMATION (per serving)

- Calories – 122

- Carbohydrate – 11g

- Protein – 4g

- Sodium – 221mg

- Potassium – 219mg

- Phosphorus – 49mg

- Dietary fiber – 2.4g

- Fat – 6g

Day #10: Baked Fish

The importance of fish is largely underestimated in the American diet. It's time to change that. This baked fish dinner recipe is super easy to follow and incredibly healthy for your kidneys.

COOKING TIME: 25 MINUTES

INGREDIENTS FOR 4 SERVINGS

SERVING SIZE: 3 oz

- Cod fillets – 1lb/0,45gr

- Olive oil – 2tbsp

- Ground cumin – ½ tsp

- Ground rosemary – ½ tsp

- Black pepper – ½ tsp

METHOD

- Preheat the oven to 350°F(176°C) and in the meantime turn cod fillet several times in olive oil, then sprinkle with spices

- Place fillets in a baking dish and bake for 20 to 25 minutes

NUTRITIONAL INFORMATION (per serving)

- Calories – 171

- Carbohydrate – 0g

- Protein – 20g

- Sodium – 69mg

- Potassium – 338mg

- Phosphorus – 204mg

- Dietary fiber – 0.2g

- Fat – 10g

Day #11: Black-Eyed Pea Hash

Peas, bell peppers, onions, and other veggies in this black-eyed pea hash deliver important nutrients for kidney health while allowing you to manage your weight. While some hash recipes are complicated, this one is simple and straightforward.

COOKING TIME: 20 MINUTES

INGREDIENTS FOR 6 SERVINGS

SERVING SIZE: 3/4 cup

- Frozen black-eyed peas (thawed) – 1 cup

- White rice (cooked) – 2 cups

- Olive oil – 1tbsp

- Garlic – 3 cloves

- Red bell pepper – 1

- Onion – 1

- Celery – 2 stalks

- Carrots – 2

- Kale – ½ cup

- Bay leaf – 1

- Fresh thyme – 3 sprigs

- Chicken broth (low-sodium) – 1 cup

- Salt – ½ tsp (optional)

- Black pepper – ¼ tsp

- Parsley – a pinch for garnish

METHOD

- Heat olive oil in a pan and add onion, garlic, celery, bell pepper, thyme, carrot, and bay leaf to sauté for 5 minutes or until fragrant

- Add peas, kale, pepper, and salt to the pan and stir before adding chicken broth.

- Add broth and then simmer for 15 minutes or until broth evaporates

- Heat rice and cover it with hash, parsley, and thyme

NUTRITIONAL INFORMATION (per serving)

- Calories – 155

- Carbohydrate – 27g

- Protein – 5g

- Sodium – 242mg

- Potassium – 318mg

- Phosphorus – 83mg

- Dietary fiber – 3g

- Fat – 3g

Day #12: Sweet Pepper, Onion, and Cabbage Combo

Cabbage, sweet pepper, and onion create a colorful and healthy combination on your plate.

COOKING TIME: 5 MINUTES

INGREDIENTS FOR 4 SERVINGS

SERVING SIZE: ½ recipe

- Green bell pepper – ½ cup

- Red bell pepper – ½ cup

- Yellow bell pepper – ½ cup

- Onion (chopped) – ½ cup

- Cabbage (shredded) – 2 cups

- White vinegar – 3tbsp

- Canola oil – 1tbsp

- Brown sugar – 1 ½ tsp

- Pepper – 1 ½ tsp

- Dijon mustard – 1 ½ tsp

METHOD

- Slice bell peppers and combine with onion, cabbage and oil in a skillet

- In a jar combine vinegar and remaining ingredients, whisk strongly and cover over vegetables

- Sauté until cabbage is tender

NUTRITIONAL INFORMATION (per serving)

- Calories – 70

- Carbohydrate – 8g

- Protein – 1g

- Sodium – 52mg

- Potassium – 208mg

- Phosphorus – 29mg

- Dietary fiber – 2g

- Fat – 4g

Day #13: Eggplant French Fries

Do you love French fries? Who doesn't, but they're not the healthiest food you can eat. Not to worry! Here's a healthy take on French fries, try it out, it's super yummy.

COOKING TIME: 5-10 MINUTES

INGREDIENTS FOR 6 SERVINGS

SERVING SIZE:7-8 pieces

- Eggplant (peeled, sliced into sticks) – 1

- Low-fat milk – 1 cup

- Eggs – 2

- Cornstarch – ¾ cup

- Unseasoned bread crumbs – ¾ cup

- Salad dressing and seasoning – 3tsp

- Hot sauce – 1tsp (optional)

- Canola oil - 1/2 cup

METHOD

- Combine milk and eggs in a bowl and add hot sauce

- In a different bowl combine cornstarch, breadcrumbs, and salad dressing or seasoning

- Heat oil over high heat and start dipping eggplant sticks in the egg mixture then coat in breadcrumbs mixture before placing into oil

- Fry for 3 minutes per batch or until eggplant fries turn golden

NUTRITIONAL INFORMATION (per serving)

- Calories – 233

- Carbohydrate – 24g

- Protein – 5g

- Sodium – 212mg

- Potassium – 215mg

- Phosphorus – 86mg

- Dietary fiber – 2.1g

- Fat – 13g

y #14: Spicy Beef Stir-Fry

This is an easy take on the classic stir-fry recipe, and it contains tender strips of beef with bell peppers, eggs, and spices.

COOKING TIME: 30-35 MINUTES

INGREDIENTS FOR 4 SERVINGS

SERVING SIZE: 1 cup

- Cornstarch – 2tbsp (separated)

- Sesame oil – ¼ tsp

- Sugar – ½ tsp

- Water – 2tbsp (separated)

- Egg (beaten) – 1

- Canola oil – 3tbsp (separated)

- Beef (sliced) – 12oz/350gr

- Green bell pepper (sliced) – 1

- Onions (sliced) – 1 cup

- Ground red chili pepper – ¼ tsp

- Sherry – 1tbsp

- Soy sauce (reduced sodium) – 2tsp

- Parsley for garnish (don't see in the method)

METHOD

- Combine one part of cornstarch, water, egg, canola oil, and beef in a bowl and marinate for 20 minutes

- Combine remainder of cornstarch and water in a different bowl

- Heat remainder of canola oil in a pan and add meat

- Cook meat until it turns brownish and adds bell pepper, chili pepper, and onion followed by sherry

- Stir-fry for 1 minute and add sesame oil, soy sauce, and sugar

- Thicken your dinner with a combination of water and cornstarch

- Before serving sprinkle with parsley

NUTRITIONAL INFORMATION (per serving)

- Calories – 261

- Carbohydrate – 10g

- Protein – 21g

- Sodium – 169mg

- Potassium – 313mg

- Phosphorus – 167mg

- Dietary fiber – 1.5g

- Fat – 15g

BONUS: Pear Salad

Dinner is the opportunity to eat something light on your stomach, and that's exactly where pear salad steps in. You've probably never tried pear in combination with cheese, but the result is outstanding.

COOKING TIME: 10-15 MINUTES

**INGREDIENTS FOR 4
SERVINGS**

SERVING SIZE: ½ cup

- Sugar – ½ cup

- Water – ½ cup

- Pecans or walnuts – ½ cup

- Lettuce – 6 cups

- Pear (peeled, diced) – 4

- Blue cheese – 2oz/60gr

- Pomegranate seeds – ½ cup

METHOD

- In a nonstick fry pan dissolve water and sugar; heat until you get a syrup-like mixture and add nuts

- Pour mixture on aluminum foil or parchment paper to separate nuts, let it cool off

- In a large bowl place lettuce where you'll add cheese, pear, and pomegranate seeds

- Before serving sprinkle with nuts and even vinegar dressing if you'd like

NUTRITIONAL INFORMATION (per serving)

- Calories – 301

- Carbohydrate – 41g

- Protein – 6g

- Sodium – 206mg

- Potassium – 297mg

- Phosphorus – 127mg

- Dietary fiber – 8.2g

- Fat – 13.7g

Chapter 8: Desserts

The renal diet does not deprive us of indulging in some delicious desserts. You just need to get a few ideas of what to make and how to prepare them. Recipes from this chapter will inspire you to make your own desserts and serve them after lunch or dinner.

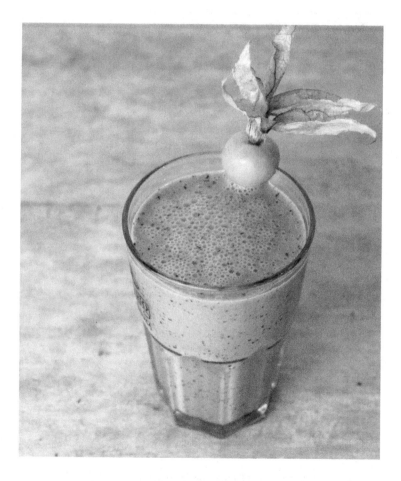

Day #1: Baked Pineapple

If you want to cook tasty and unique dessert, this recipe is absolutely right choice. This dessert is perfect for any time of the year.

COOKING TIME: 30 MINUTES

INGREDIENTS FOR 9 SERVINGS

SERVING SIZE: ½ cup

- Pineapple with juice – 20oz/570gr

- Eggs – 2

- Sugar – 2 cups

- Tapioca – 3tbsp

- Salt – 1/8 tsp

- Unsalted butter – 3tbsp

- Cinnamon – ½ tsp

METHOD

- First, preheat the oven to 350°F (176°C)

- Combine pineapple with eggs, sugar, tapioca, and salt in a bowl

- Pour mixture into a baking dish (8"x8")

- Place butter slices on top of the mixture and sprinkle with cinnamon, bake for 30 minutes

NUTRITIONAL INFORMATION (per serving)

- Calories – 270

- Carbohydrate – 54g

- Protein – 2g

- Sodium – 50mg

- Potassium – 85mg

- Phosphorus – 26mg

- Dietary fiber – 0.6g

- Fat – 5g

Day #2: Blueberry Smoothie

Blueberries are an abundant source of vitamins and antioxidants that protect us in more ways than one. This smoothie is delicious and looks pretty, meaning it's also a great dessert to serve when you're in a hurry.

COOKING TIME: 2 MINUTES

> **INGREDIENTS FOR 3 SERVINGS**

SERVING SIZE: 1 cup

- Frozen blueberries (slightly thawed) – 2 cups

- Pineapple juice – 1 ¼ cup

- Egg whites – ¾ cup

- Splendid or sugar – 2tsp

- Water – ½ cup

METHOD

- Combine all ingredients in a blender and puree

- Serve

NUTRITIONAL INFORMATION (per serving)

- Calories – 155.4

- Carbohydrate – 31.1g

- Protein – 7.4g

- Sodium – 104.1mg

- Potassium – 289.4mg

- Phosphorus – 27.5mg

- Dietary fiber – 3g

- Fat – 0.75mg

Day #3: Fried Apples

Apple is one of the most accessible fruits in the world, and that's why they make such a great dessert choice. Cinnamon and vanilla give this dessert a warm and tasty scent and a dose of deliciousness, of course.

COOKING TIME: 5-10 MINUTES

INGREDIENTS FOR 5 SERVINGS

SERVING SIZE: ½ apple

- Apples (peeled, sliced) – 5 cups

- Vanilla – 1tsp

- Cinnamon – 2tsp

METHOD

- Coat skillet with a cooking spray and add apples

- Sauté apples until soft and sprinkle with cinnamon and vanilla

NUTRITIONAL INFORMATION (per serving)

- Calories – 94

- Carbohydrate – 1g

- Protein – 0g

- Sodium – 1g

- Potassium – 153mg

- Phosphorus – 10mg

- Dietary fiber – 5.9g

- Fat – 0.4g

Day #4: Chia Pudding with Berries

Chia seeds may be tiny, but they hold an enormous health potential. The best thing about them is that you can add these seeds to a wide spectrum of recipes. Berries and chia are a perfect combination.

COOKING TIME: 60 MINUTES

INGREDIENTS FOR 4 SERVINGS

SERVING SIZE: ½ cup plus berries

- Almond milk – 1 cup

- Chia seeds – ½ cup

- Coconut (sweetened, shredded) – ¼ cup

- Blueberries – ¼ cup

- Strawberries – 4

METHOD

- Blend chia seeds and almond milk together and pour the mixture into dessert dishes

158

- Refrigerate mixture for an hour (or 30 minutes in the freezer)

- When serving, sprinkle with coconut, strawberry, and blueberries

NUTRITIONAL INFORMATION (per serving)

- Calories – 184

- Carbohydrate – 22g

- Protein – 4g

- Sodium – 94mg

- Potassium – 199mg

- Phosphorus – 200mg

- Dietary fiber – 8g

- Fat – 9g

Day #5: Simple and Easy Pumpkin Cheesecake

Simple and easy pumpkin cheesecake takes the hassle out of the whole process and gives us the opportunity to make delicious dessert even if our culinary skills aren't on the highest level. This is an ideal dessert for the fall season.

COOKING TIME: 55 MINUTES

INGREDIENTS FOR 8 SERVINGS

SERVING SIZE: 1/8 pie

- 9" pie crust – 1

- Egg white – 1

- Cream cheese – 16oz/455gr

- Granulated sugar – ½ cup

- Vanilla extract – 1tsp

- Egg substitute – ½ cup

- Pumpkin puree – ½ cup

160

- Pumpkin pie spice – 1tsp

- Frozen dessert topping – 8tbsp

METHOD

- Preheat the oven to 375°F(190°C)

- Use egg white to brush pie crust and bake for 5 minutes then decrease the heat to 350°F(176°C)

- Combine sugar, cheese, and vanilla in a bowl and mix thoroughly, then add egg substitute followed by pumpkin spice and puree

- Pour the mixture into pie crust and bake for 40 to 50 minutes, let it cool before putting the pie in the fridge

- Slice into eight pieces and serve with one tablespoon of dessert topping

NUTRITIONAL INFORMATION (per serving)

- Calories – 365

- Carbohydrate – 29g

- Protein – 6g

- Sodium – 245mg

- Potassium – 126mg

- Phosphorus – 66mg

- Dietary fiber – 0.7g

- Fat – 25g

Day #6: Microwave Lemon Curd

Microwave lemon curd can serve as a filling, and you can also add it to pie crusts and use it in many other ways. The best thing about this simple recipe is that you can make it in batches and use it when necessary or store up to three weeks.

COOKING TIME: 10-20 MINUTES

> **INGREDIENTS FOR 16 SERVINGS**

SERVING SIZE: 1 tbsp

- Granulated sugar – 1 cup

- Eggs – 3

- Lemon juice – 2/3 cup

- Lemons (zested) – 3

- Butter (melted) – ½ cup

METHOD

- Combine sugar and eggs in a microwave-safe bowl and add lemon juice and zest, and butter

- Cook the mixture in the microwave in intervals of one minute, stirring and returning back to microwave until it's done

- Pour the mixture into jars

NUTRITIONAL INFORMATION (per serving)

- Calories – 115

- Carbohydrate – 14g

- Protein – 1g

- Sodium – 54mg

- Potassium – 28mg

- Phosphorus – 20mg

- Dietary fiber – 0.3g

- Fat – 6.7g

Day #7: Frozen Fruit Delight

If you are looking for a dessert that will revitalize you, boost energy levels, and be good to your kidneys, then this is the one. Frozen fruit delight is particularly delicious during hot summer days and nights.

COOKING TIME: 2-3 HOURS

> **INGREDIENTS FOR 10 SERVINGS**

SERVING SIZE: ½ cup

- Cherries – 1/3 cup

- Crushed pineapple – 8oz/230gr

- Sour cream (reduced fat) – 8oz/230gr

- Lemon juice – 1tbsp

- Strawberries (sliced) – 1 cup

- Sugar – ½ cup

- Salt – 1/8 tsp

- Whipped topping – 3 cups

METHOD

- Drain pineapple and chop cherries

- Combine all ingredients except whipped topping and blend until smooth.

- Then, add whipped topping

- Put the mixture in a container and freeze for 2 to 3 hours or until it hardens

NUTRITIONAL INFORMATION (per serving)

- Calories – 133

- Carbohydrate – 21g

- Protein – 1g

- Sodium – 59mg

- Potassium – 99mg

- Phosphorus – 36mg

- Dietary fiber – 0.8g

- Fat – 5g

Day #8: No-Bake Peanut Butter Balls

Chances are you have peanut butter in your kitchen as well as cream cheese and chocolate chips. Make these kidney-friendly peanut butter balls to treat yourself with a nice and stress-free dessert.

COOKING TIME: 1 HOUR

INGREDIENTS FOR 12 SERVINGS

SERVING SIZE: 1 ball

- Peanut butter (unsalted, unsweetened) – ½ cup

- Cream cheese (reduced fat) – 8oz

- Graham cracker crumbs – 1 ¼ cups

- Mini chocolate chips – ¼ cup

- Vanilla – 1tsp

- Coconut (shredded) – ½ cup (optional)

METHOD

- Combine all ingredients except coconut and blend them

- Start rolling dough into 1-inch balls

- Roll balls into shredded coconut

- Put in the fridge for about an hour

NUTRITIONAL INFORMATION (per serving)

- Calories – 150

- Carbohydrate – 13g

- Protein – 4g

- Sodium – 120mg

- Potassium – 106mg

- Phosphorus – 65mg

- Dietary fiber – 1.5g

- Fat – 11.7g

Day #9: Fresh Fruit Compote

Fresh fruit compote is one of the easiest desserts you can make. Whether you like it warm or cold, this dessert is always delicious.

COOKING TIME: 5 MINUTES

INGREDIENTS FOR 8 SERVINGS

SERVING SIZE: ½ cup

Cooking time: 5 minutes

Serving size: 8

Ingredients:

- Strawberries – ½ cup

- Blackberries – ½ cup

- Blueberries – ½ cup

- Peach – ½ cup

- Red raspberry – ¼ cup

- Orange juice – ½ cup

- Apple (diced) – 1

- Banana (diced) - 1

METHOD

- Pour orange juice into a container and add all ingredients

- Gently toss to combine

NUTRITIONAL INFORMATION (per serving)

- Calories – 44

- Carbohydrate – 11g

- Protein – 0.5g

- Sodium – 1mg

- Potassium – 140mg

- Phosphorus – 13mg

- Dietary fiber – 1.6g

- Fat – 0.2g

Day #10: Ambrosia

Ambrosia is yet another dessert you don't have to bake. Just follow simple instructions, combine fruits and other ingredients, and your delicious dessert is ready.

COOKING TIME: 1 HOUR

INGREDIENTS FOR 12 SERVINGS

SERVING SIZE: ½ cup

- Sour cream – 1 cup

- Powdered sugar – ½ cup

- Vanilla extract – ½ tsp

- Pineapple chunks – 15oz/430gr

- Peaches (sliced) – 15oz/430gr

- Cherries – 1 ½ cup

- Marshmallows – 3 cups

- Lettuce leaves - 12

METHOD

- Combine sour cream, sugar, and vanilla, then add cherries, peaches, marshmallow, and pineapple

- Stir gently

- Let sit in the fridge for an hour

- Serve on lettuce leaves

NUTRITIONAL INFORMATION (per serving)

- Calories – 176

- Carbohydrate – 36g

- Protein – 1g

- Sodium – 17mg

- Potassium – 132mg

- Phosphorus – 28mg

- Dietary fiber – 1.1g

- Fat – 4g

Day #11: Mango Smoothie

Smoothies are simple, nutrient-dense, and they have a divine texture. This mango smoothie is an ideal dessert, regardless of the time of the day.

COOKING TIME: 2 MINUTES

INGREDIENTS FOR 2 SERVINGS

SERVING SIZE: 1 cup

- Plain yogurt – 1 cup

- Milk – ½ cup

- Mango juice – ½ cup

- Sugar – 1-3tbsp

- Cardamom – ¼ tsp

- Lime juice – ¼ cup (optional)

METHOD

- Blend all ingredients in a food processor or blender for 2 minutes

- Serve

NUTRITIONAL INFORMATION (per serving)

- Calories – 169

- Carbohydrate – 29g

- Protein – 9g

- Sodium – 143mg

- Potassium – 98mg

- Phosphorus – 59mg

- Dietary fiber – 0.1g

- Fat – 2.8g

Day #12: Bagel Bread Pudding

Here's a useful suggestion for a delicious dessert you can make if you have leftover bread.

COOKING TIME: 30 MINUTES

INGREDIENTS FOR 4 SERVINGS

SERVING SIZE: ¼ recipe

- Bagels – 2

- Liquid nondairy creamer – 2

- Egg substitute – ½ cup

- Sugar – ½ cup

- Cinnamon – 1tsp

METHOD

- Using a cooking spray coat a baking dish where you will place bagel chopped into small pieces

- Mix other ingredients and pour over bread, let sit a few minutes until liquid is absorbed

- Bake 30 minutes or until bread is brownish in an oven set to 350°F(176°C)

NUTRITIONAL INFORMATION (per serving)

- Calories – 310

- Carbohydrate – 52g

- Protein – 8g

- Sodium – 281mg

- Potassium – 169mg

- Phosphorus – 99mg

- Dietary fiber – 1.3g

- Fat – 7g

Day #13: Lemon and Ginger Cookies

Lemon and ginger cookies are a wonderful alternative to "regular" cookies that most people love. The baking process is easy, and cookies taste heavenly.

COOKING TIME: 52 MINUTES

INGREDIENTS FOR 12 SERVINGS

SERVING SIZE: 2 cookies

- Butter (unsalted) – ½ cup

- Sugar – ½ cup

- Egg – 1

- Baking soda – ½ tsp

- Lemon juice – 2tbsp

- Lemon zest – 1tbsp

- Ginger (fresh, peeled, chopped) – 1tbsp

- Flour – 1 ¼ cups

- Toasted coconut (unsweetened) – 1 cup

METHOD

- Preheat the oven to 350°F(176°C), pour coconut on the baking sheet and bake 5 to 10 minutes or until brown

- Remove coconut from an oven into a bowl and set aside

- Combine butter and sugar with a mixer until fluffy, then add lemon juice, egg, lemon zest, ginger and mix again

- Combine flour and baking soda with butter mixture, mix thoroughly and let alone for 30 minutes

- Make balls out of dough and place them on the baking sheet, bake for 10 to 12 minutes

NUTRITIONAL INFORMATION (per serving)

- Calories – 97

- Carbohydrate – 11g

- Protein – 1g

- Sodium – 40mg

- Potassium – 27mg

- Phosphorus – 17mg

- Dietary fiber – 0.4g

- Fat – 6g

Day #14: Milk-Free Hot Cocoa

Childhood days are long gone, but it doesn't mean we shouldn't indulge in a nice cup of hot cocoa. This healthy alternative will blow your mind.

COOKING TIME: 5 MINUTES

INGREDIENTS FOR 1 SERVING

SERVING SIZE: 1 cup

- Hot water – 1 cup

- Unsweetened cocoa powder – 1tbsp

- Sugar – 2tsp

- Coldwater – 2tbsp

- Whipped dessert topping – 3tbsp

METHOD

- To hot water add sugar and cocoa powder, then combine with cold water and form a paste-like mixture

- Add hot water into the cup and stir

- Serve with whipped dessert topping

NUTRITIONAL INFORMATION (per serving)

- Calories – 72

- Carbohydrate – 13g

- Protein – 1g

- Sodium – 10mg

- Potassium – 100mg

- Phosphorus – 49mg

- Dietary fiber – 1.8g

- Fat – 3g

BONUS: Chinese Sponge Cakes

Chinese sponge cake is an ideal dessert solution for situations when you want to eat something delicious, but not in the mood to go to the store to buy some ingredients for more demanding cakes and treats.

COOKING TIME: 40 MINUTES

**INGREDIENTS FOR 4
SERVING**

SERVING SIZE: 1 piece

- Eggs – 2

- Sugar – ½ cup

- Vanilla – ½ tsp

- Flour – ½ cup

- Baking powder – ¼ tsp

METHOD
- Preheat the oven to 325°F(162°C) and fill a pan with water and place it into the oven

- Use a parchment paper to line four custard cups

- Beat eggs and add sugar, vanilla, flour, and baking powder

- Pour mixture into lined custard cups and place into the pan filled with water in the oven

- Cook for 30 minutes or until a knife comes out clean when you insert it

NUTRITIONAL INFORMATION (per serving)

- Calories – 194

- Carbohydrate – 37g

- Protein – 5g

- Sodium – 62mg

- Potassium – 50mg

- Phosphorus – 67mg

- Dietary fiber – 0.4g

- Fat – 2.6g

Chapter 9: FAQs About Dialysis and How to Avoid It

In 2016, the last year for which data is available, about 125,000 people in the United States started treatment for end-stage kidney disease (ESKD), and over 726,000 were on dialysis. In other words, two in 1000 people in the US were on a dialysis[2]. The last chapter of this book is reserved for the most common questions about dialysis and tips to avoid it.

What is Dialysis?

Dialysis is a treatment to remove waste products and excess fluids from the blood when kidneys do not work properly. The procedure is done in the hospital, a dialysis unit that is not part of the hospital, or even in a patient's home.

Who Needs dialysis?

Dialysis is recommended to patients who develop ESKD by the time they lose 85% to 90% of their kidney function. In other words, doctors recommend dialysis when only 10% to 15% of the kidneys are functional in order to help them expel waste and excess fluid when they are unable to do it on their own.

What are the Types of Dialysis?

There are two types of dialysis:

- Hemodialysis – revolves around diverting blood into the external machine, which filters it and then returns the blood to the body. The machine acts as an artificial kidney and returns the blood without salts, wastes, and excess fluid. Most patients need hemodialysis three times a week for four hours per treatment

- Peritoneal dialysis – includes pumping dialysis fluid into the patient's peritoneum, located in the abdomen, to draw out waste products

Can I Do Dialysis on My Own?

Yes, there is a self-care dialysis option where a patient can learn to do some or complete dialysis treatment. Self-care dialysis offers more flexibility, independence, and reduces waiting times. For more information about self-dialysis, you should consult your healthcare provider.

What to Expect During Dialysis Treatment?

Bear in mind that dialysis treatment lasts for hours, every time. Make sure you plan and organize your day accordingly. Many patients bring a book or magazine.

What are the Side Effects of Dialysis?

Not every patient experiences adverse reactions to dialysis, but those who do may have side effects such as fatigue, cramping, stress and anxiety, hernia, loss of libido, itchy skin, sepsis, and low blood pressure.

Do I Need to Quit My Job?

Many patients on dialysis still have their job. Of course, it is important to adjust the work schedule to the dialysis appointments. People who do physical labor may need to make some changes.

How to Avoid Dialysis?

Not every patient with kidney disease needs dialysis. It's entirely possible to reduce the risk and avoid dialysis by adherence to doctor-recommended treatment and lifestyle adjustments. In order to avoid dialysis, you should eat a renal diet, lose weight or maintain it in a healthy range, quit smoking, control blood pressure, manage diabetes, see your doctor regularly, treat UTIs properly.

Conclusion

Once again, I would like to thank you for purchasing this book. Now that we have come to an end you are probably inspired to start cooking delicious meals to support kidney health.

As seen throughout this cookbook, following a kidney-friendly diet is not the most difficult task in the world.

Recipes from this cookbook are simple, delicious, and healthy. You can even use them as an inspiration to experiment and create your own renal diet recipes. Options are truly endless.

Bear in mind that the renal diet is a lifestyle, and to get the best results, it's important to follow it regularly and include it in your daily life. And don't worry, you can do it. After all, this book is the best proof that the renal diet is yummy. Meals do not require too much hassle, and that's also amazing.

If you liked the book feel free to rate and review it. That would help other people with kidney disease to get this cookbook and manage their condition more effectively.

Start cooking and experimenting with these recipes today.

You'll love it.

Please always consult with your family doctor or nutritionist before using a current recipe or the diet program.

Thanks for your attention!

Made in the USA
Monee, IL
14 March 2020